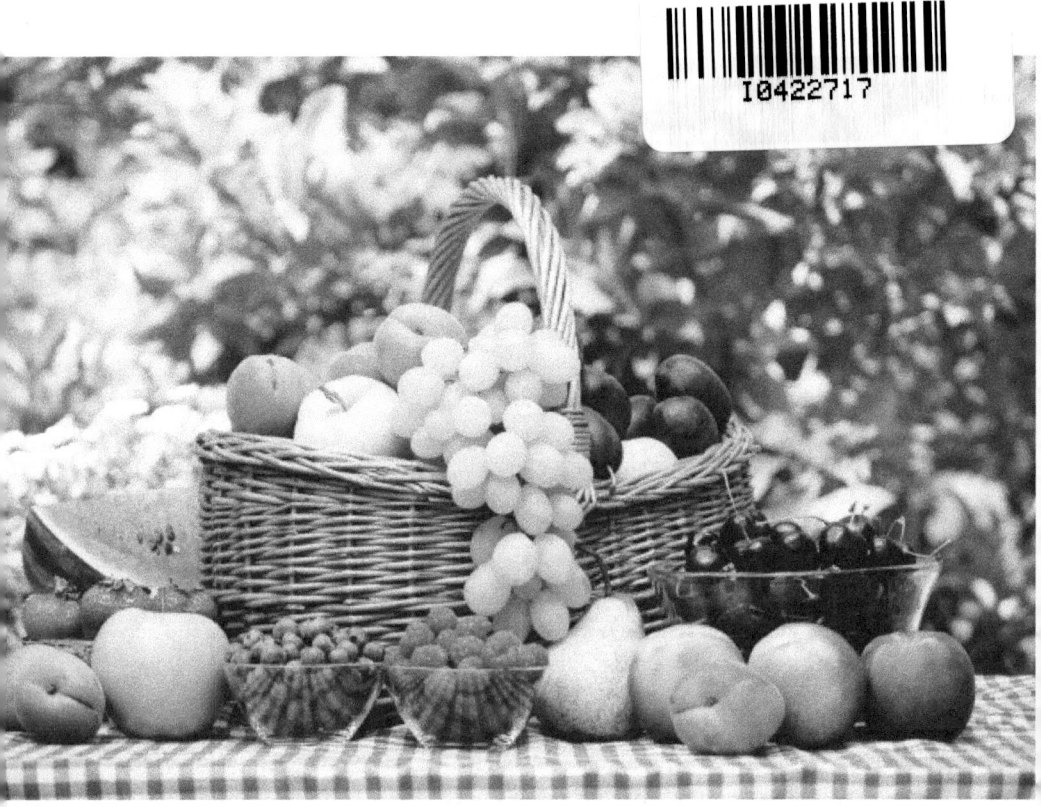

Body Foods 1

Ommey Salma Shammi

In the name of ALLAH

ALLAH has created so many foods for us and given us knowledge to pick the best.

This is my first book, I hope people will get benefited by reading this book.

This book is about food. Some foods are healthy and some are unhealthy. So this book will help to give general idea about healthy and unhealthy food. We have lots of food surround us and some of these provide us vitamin, mineral, nutrients, fiber and energy to keep us healthy, fit, fight against disease and give us energy and some of these are unhealthy and provide us toxins, carcinogen agents and causing diseases. Some foods are beneficial , on the other hand some can be harmful and every time it is hard to keep remember about their effect on the body. But if we become used to about the foods in our daily routine which benefits us, then it is easy to remember them and discards the food that harmful for our body system and cause diseases. The body will reflects what we eat. So be careful and wise about daily food routine especially with the ageing process. At one point our body's metabolism system become slow, so then it is very important to avoid harmful and junk foods, select proper foods, choose right amount of food and right foods beneficial for our body system, immune system and keep all the system healthy

Content:

Acne

Aging process

Arthritis

Skin

Cancer

Cardiovascular Health

Diabetes

Eczema/Atopic dermatitis

Gout

Psoriasis

Immune System

Inflammation

Irritable bowel syndrome

Kidney disease

Brain health

Reproductive Health

Menopausal symptom

Premenstrual tension (PMT)

Sleeping problem

Stress

Urinary problem

Vitiligo

Weight

Acne:

Foods help to reduce acne

Avocado:

- Treat acne naturally
- Rich in vitamin C

Artichoke:

- Good source of antioxidants and vitamin C
- Helps to remove toxin from body

Broccoli:

- Packed with vitamins A, B complex and K
- Helps to clear skin

Brown Rice:

- Packed with vitamin B, protein, magnesium, and several antioxidants

Dark chocolate:

- It has anti oxidants

Fatty fishes:

- Omega 3 and 6 fatty acids fight against acne

Fennel:

- Improve digestion
- natural skin cleanser

Flax seeds:

- Omega 3 fatty acid helps to improve acne

Garlic:

- Fight against inflammation

Green tea:

- Rich in antioxidants
- Helps to relief skin stress

Nuts:

- Contain selenium, vitamin E, copper, magnesium, manganese, potassium, calcium and iron,
- Helpful for healthy skin

Pumpkin/Pumpkin seed:

- Helps in treating acne

Radish:

- Clear skin

Red grapes:

- Rich in antioxidants
- Reduce inflammation of skin

Sweet potato:

- Low glycemic-index, no effect on blood sugar level
- Improve skin health

Spinach:

- It cleans the toxin from the body

Whole grain:

- Low glycemic-index, no effect on blood sugar level
- Improve skin health

Yogurt :

- Good for healthy skin

Foods increase acne:

(If you find any relation with any specific food, then it is better to avoid, but acne is usually not related to food)

Cow's milk:

- Increase insulin which increase skin oil production

Deep fried food:

- Cause inflammation

Fast food:

- Cause inflammation

Processed food:

- Cereals, white bread, white rice, pretzels, potato chips, cookies, cake

- Packed with calorie and sugar

- It can cause break out of skin and related to cause acne

Aging process:

Foods slow down aging process:

Asparagus:

- Very high in antioxidants
- Neutralize free radicals
- Also helps to slow the ageing process

Avocados:

- Loaded with Vitamins and healthy fats
- Flush harmful toxins from the body

Blueberries:

- High in vitamin C
- helps in smooth and clean skin

Carrots:

- High in vitamin A (beta carotene)
- Clear skin and produce collagen
- Remove free radicals which damage skin

Green tea:

- Contain polyphenol antioxidants, protects from sun radiation
- High in vitamin c helps collagen formation

Honey:

- Can be added with green tea which benefits skin

Nuts:

- Contain omega 3 fatty acid, helps skin to be healthy and glow

Olive oil:

- Helps skin to be healthy

Peaches:

- Rich in vitamin C, A, K ; magnesium and potassium
- Protect against harmful UV rays
- Reduce free radicals
- Remove dark circle under eyes
- Regenerate skin collagen tissue

Pomegranate:

- Contained antioxidants
- Stop production of free radicals
- Prevent wrinkle
- Repair cell damage

Raspberries:

- Contain phytochemicals, which help slow down aging process

Salmon :

- Rich in protein and essential fatty acids, vitamins and minerals
- Protect against macular degeneration (an eye disease, causes of blindness with age)

Strawberries:

- High in photochemical that slow down the signs of ageing

Yogurt:

- Delay facial wrinkle

Foods faster aging process:

Margarine:

- Contain bad fat (trans fat)
- Faster the wrinkle appear

Microwave dinner:

- Frozen meals high in sodium

Energy drinks:

- No nutrients
- High sugar which faster the wrinkle

Baked food:

- Often high in sugar and fat

Sausage:

- Preservatives used in processed meats which fasten the ageing

Corn syrup

- Sugar damage the skin collagen

Sugary cocktails

- Contain High sugar

Sugar:

- Cause inflammation
- Damage skin collagen and elastin

High glycemic index carbs

- Bagels, oatmeal, pretzels, pasta, and cereal,
- Accelerate the skin's aging process
- Causing acne and rosacea

Alcohol:

- Dehydrate skin
- Make fine lines and wrinkles more

High Salt foods

- Retain water and feel bloated

Deep fried food

- These food damage both inside and outside
- Free radical damage the skin

Agave:

- These sweet syrup contain high fructose
- Breaks down collagen
- Making fine lines more appear

Candy:

- Cause weight gain
- Contain processed sugar

Charcoal meat:

- Any meat that is blackened is very bad for body
- Cause infection
- Break down collagen
- Faster ageing process

Potato chips:

- Contain bad fats or oil
- Down body immune system

Pepperoni Pizza:

- Processed meats cause inflammation

Arthritis:

Foods benefit in Arthritis:

Asparagus

Beets

Broccoli

Carrot

Cauliflower

Celery seeds

Cherries

Extra virgin olive oil

Flaxseeds

Garlic

Ginger

Mangoes

onions

Papayas

Rosemary

Sesame seeds

Sunflower oil

Turmeric

Foods that harm Arthritis:

Blackened or barbeque food

Eggplant

Fast foods

French fries

Gluten (bagels, bread, pasta)

Pepper

Potatoes

Tobacco

Tomatoes

Skin

Foods Keep skin beautiful

Avocado

Dark chocolate

Eggplant

Eggs

Green tea :

- Rich in antioxidants and vitamins
- protect from sun radiation and helps to form collagen

Lemon:

- High in vitamin C which helps to build collagen

Oatmeal

Radish:

- Rich in vitamins and minerals
- Maintain healthy moisture in skin
- Clear up skin
- Reduce rash, crack

Soy

Flaxseed:

- Grind them and then add to recipe

Sunflower seeds

Walnut:

- Delay the process of ageing

Water:

- Drink 6-8 glasses of water everyday
- Flush the toxin from the body

Yoghurt

Foods that harm skin

Agave:

- Sweet syrups made from speed up wrinkle

Candy:

- Processed sugar cause harm

Cereal:

- Many cereals are refined and packed with added sugar, cause wrinkle

Chips:

- Refined carbohydrate cause wrinkle, fine line

Deli meat:

- It can cause wrinkle

Fast food:

- Cause blemishes

Frozen Yogurt

Juice:

- Added sugar cause premature skin ageing

Margarine:

- Contain trans fat, increase wrinkle
- Decrease hydration of the body

Milk:

- It is good for body but has some negativity on skin
- It can cause acne

Processed food

Rice cake:

- Speed up wrinkle

Sherbet:

- Added sugar cause premature skin ageing

Soda:

- Cause premature skin ageing

Cancer

Food fight against cancer:

Apples:

- Contain soluble fiber
- Fight against breast and colon cancer

Blueberiies:

- High in antioxidants, phytochemicals and flavonoids
- Reduce risk of cancer

Broccoli

- Inhibit the growth of cancer cell
- Reduce production of free radicals

Brussels sprouts

- Inhibit the growth of cancer cell
- Reduce production of free radicals

Cabbage

- High in vitamin K, C, fiber
- Good source of vitamin B6 and folic acid.
- Contain phytochemicals (usually found in fruits and vegetables)
- Inhibit the growth of cancer cell
- Reduce production of free radicals

Cauliflower

- Inhibit the growth of cancer cell
- Reduce production of free radicals

Cranberries

- High in vitamin C and D; potassium, iron
- Raw cranberries fight against cancer

Flax seed:

- Rich source of lignan, a powerful antioxidants
- Fight against cancer , especially breast cancer

Goji berries/ wolfberries:

- Rich in vitamin A and antioxidants
- Help to protect from skin cancer
- Benefit immune system

Grapefruits:

- Though high in fiber, pectin
- Rich in vitamin c
- Contain phytonutrients, fight against cancer

Kale

- Inhibit the growth of cancer cell
- Reduce production of free radicals

Mango:

- Helps to protects against skin cancer

Oranges:

- Rich in vitamin, mineral, antioxidants and folate
- Cancer fighter
- Immune booster

Pak choi

- Inhibit the growth of cancer cell
- Reduce production of free radicals

Papaya:

- Rich in vitamin, mineral, antioxidants and folate
- **Fight against colon cancer, lung cancer**

Peppers:

- Packed with phytochemicals
- High in vitamin C and A.
- Neutralize free radicals in the body which damage the cell
- Prevent cancer

Pomegranate:

- Reduce the prostate cancer

Pumpkin:

- Rich in fiber, beta carotene (vitamin A)
- Reduce risk of lung cancer

Radish:

- Act as a detoxifier, eliminate toxin and waste from the body
- Helps to fight against the cancer

Raspberries:

- High in photochemical that fight against cancer

Spinach:

- Contain powerful antioxidants, high amount iron, calcium and oxalate compound
- Fight against cancers especially breast, colon and ovarian.

Spirulina:

- Green algae (found in salt water lake)
- Rich in vitamin B, calcium, iron
- reduce tiredness
- fight against cancer and infection

Strawberries:

- High in photochemical that fight against cancer

Walnut:

- Fight against cancer especially breast cancer

Foods that cause Cancer:

Alcohol:

- One of the leading cause of cancer

Canned tomatoes:

- Contain chemical lined in the canned
- Can cause cancer, heart disease and reproductive problem

Farm raised Salmon:

- Contaminated with chemicals, antibiotics, pesticide and other cancer causing agents

GMO (Genetically Modified Foods):

- Most of the corn and soy are genetically modified

Microwave popcorn:

- The bag is lined with cancer causing chemicals
- Risks for liver, testicular and pancreatic cancer

Potato chips:

- Contain bad fat, artificial flavors and excess salt

Processed meat:

- Deli meats contain excess salt and chemical
- Risk for cancer

Processed food:

- Any salty, pickled and smoked food increase the risk of cancer

Red meat:

- Every day in diet may increase the risk of cancer

Soft drinks:

- Full of calorie, sugar and no nutrients

Sugar:

- Any refined sugar, artificial sweeteners increase risk of cancer

Vegetable oil:

- It extracted by chemically

Cardiovascular health

(Cardiovascular system includes heart, blood vessels and blood flow)

Foods benefit cardiovascular health

Apple:

- Packed with vitamins, fiber and minerals
- Reduce blood pressure

Avocados:

- High in fiber and good fats

Beets:

- Packed with vitamin C, fiber and nutrients
- Protect against cancer, heart disease, and inflammation

Blueberries:

- High in antioxidants, phytochemicals and flavonoids
- Reduce bad cholesterol

Chickpeas:

- Rich in vitamin B6
- Help reduce premenstrual tension

Cinnamon:

- Increase blood flow through the body

Coconut oil:

- Excellent to use as cooking oil
- Absorbed quickly and easily by the body
- Burn more fat

- Lower cholesterol slightly
- Protect against heart disease

Cranberries:

- Improve blood cholesterol

Dark chocolate/raw cacao :

- Rich in antioxidants
- Dairy free 70% or higher improves blood flow,
- Lower blood pressure and bad cholesterol

Flaxseeds:

- Lower blood cholesterol
- Reduce heart attack

Garlic:

- Reduce bad cholesterol

Green tea:

- Very high in antioxidants
- Thought to help fat burning
-

Oats:

- High in fibre and vitamin B
- Lower the cholesterol

Olive oil:

- High in oleic acid
- Helps to keep cardiovascular system healthy

Onions:

- Rich in antioxidants
- Lower the cholesterol

Papaya:

- Rich in vitamin, mineral, antioxidants and folate
- Fight against heart disease
- Control heart rate and blood pressure

Pomegranate:

- Prevent heart disease
- Unclog arteries

Pumpkin:

- Rich in fiber, beta carotene (vitamin A)
- Prevent high blood pressure

Radish:

- It relax vessels and improve blood flow
- Helps to reduce blood pressure

Spinach:

- Contain powerful antioxidants, high amount iron, calcium and oxalate compound
- Protect the heart from cardiovascular disease.

Sweet Potatoes:

- Rich in beta carotene, antioxidants, vitamin C and B6
- May prevent clogged arteries

Quinoa:

- High in fiber, nutrients, iron, copper, magnesium
- Contain all the essential amino acid to make a complete protein

- Reduce frequency of migraine
- Reduce risk high blood pressure and heart attack

Walnut:

- Rich in omega 3 fatty acids
- Improve cholesterol and blood pressure

Watercress:
- Rich in vitamin K and antioxidants
- Prevent hardening of arteries

Foods harm cardiovascular health

Alcohol

Bacon and sausage

Beef jerky

Blended coffee

Burgers

Canned vegetables

Cheese

Cheesecake

Chinese take out

Cinnamon rolls

Coffee cream

Cottage cheese

Fast food

Fat, margarine

French fries

Fried chicken

Frozen meals

Fruit juice

Ice cream

Ketchup

Potato chips

Processed food(Cake, cookies, pizza, pasta, biscuits)

Processed meat

Red meat

Restaurant soup

Salt

Soda

Steak

Sugar

Tomato sauce

Vegetable sauce

White rice

Diabetes:

Foods helpful in Diabetes:

Almond

Apples:

Asparagus

Avocados

Bean

Berries

Bitter melon

Broccoli

Carrot

Cinnamon:

- Stabilize blood sugar levels
- Increase blood flow through the body

Egg white

Fish

Flaxseeds

Green tea

Melons:

- Watermelon, honeydew, rockmelon

Nuts

Oat meal

Olive oil

Radish:

- Does not impact on blood sugar level
- Helps to absorb sugar from the blood

Red grapefruit

Red onion

Spinach :

- Contain powerful antioxidants, high amount iron, calcium and oxalate compound

Sweet potatoes

Tomatoes

Turkey:

- Helps in blood-sugar regulation.

Foods To Be Avoided in Diabetes:

Artificial Sweeteners,

Cakes And Pastries

coffee

Energy Drinks,

French Fries,

Fruit Juices,

Palm oil

Potatoes,

Raisins,

Red Meat

Soft Drinks,

White Bread,

White Rice

Whole Milk

Eczema/Atopic dermatitis

Eczema is common in children under 2 years of age, but can affect older children and adults. Many people diagnosed with eczema also have food allergies.

Food benefits in eczema:

Apples:

- Contains quercetin to lower histamine

Banana:

- Contain histamine lowering agent, magnesium and vitamin C.

Beef/Chicken broth:

- skin-repairing amino acid glycine.

Blueberries:

- Contains quercetin to lower histamine

Broccoli

- Contains quercetin to lower histamine:

Buckwheat:

- Gluten-free and contains quercetin to lower histamine and has strong anti-inflammatory effect

Fatty fish:

- Contain omega 3 fatty acid

Green onions:

- Contain histamine-lowering, anti-inflammatory quercetin
- Rich source of vitamin K
- Important for healthy skin.

Kale

Miso soup

Olive oil

Potato:

- Rich in fibre, potassium, vitamin C and is alkalizing.

Radish:

- Reduce skin allergy, rash and cracks

Rice milk:

- Low allergy and low in chemicals and considered eczema safe

Spinach

Walnut

Some foods involve with allergy and eczema are:

Cow's milk

Egg

Fish

Gluten

Nut

Shellfish

Soy product

Gout:

Foods Helpful:

Normal well balance diet,

Foods to Avoid:

Alcohol,

Sugar

Soft drinks,

Organ meats- Liver, brain, kidneys, sweetbread

Shellfish and game,

Tinned fish-sardines, anchovies, herrings

Lifestyle:

Good fluid intake

Weight reduction

Factor:

Avoid drugs-diuretics, salicylate, low dose aspirin

Psoriasis:

Foods Helpful:

Apples,

Apricots,

Blueberries

Carrots,

Cucumbers,

Extra virgin oilve oil,

Flax seeds,

Lentils, kale,

Mangoes,

Papayas,

Pars,

Pumpkin seeds,

Pumpkin,

Sesame seeds,

Spinach,

Strawberries, oats,

Sunflower seeds,

Watercress

Foods Avoid:

Sugar,

Alcohol,

Artificial sweeteners,

Fried foods,

Soft drinks,

Refined sugar

Lifestyle:

Avoid sunburn, emotional stress, trauma or physical stress,

Factor

Drugs-NSAIDs, Oral contraceptive, lithium, Beta blocker, choloquine.

Immune system:

Immune system booster foods:

Almonds:

- Rich in vitamin E and healthy fats
- Prevent and fight against infection

Banana:

- Contain cytolcin which may help to increase white blood cell
- Strengthen immune system
- Reduce stress

Broccoli:

- Packed with vitamins A, C and E.
- Rich in antioxidants and fiber

Citrus fruits:

Clementine, Grape, Lemons, Lime, Oranges, Tangerines

- Rich with vitamin C
- Build up immune system
- Thought to increase white blood cells
- Fight infection

Cranberries:

- High in vitamins C, D; potassium, iron
- Boost immunity and protect against cancer

Dark chocolate:

- Boost immune system

Egg:

- High in protein and vitamin D
- Protect and boost immune system

Garlic:

- Contain sulfur compound (allicin)
- Fight against infection
- Slow down hardening of arteries
- lower blood pressure

Ginger:

- Reduce inflammation
- Decrease chronic pain
- May help lower cholesterol

Goji berries/ wolfberries:

- Rich in vitamin A and antioxidants
- Help to protect from skin cancer
- Benefit immune system

Green tea :

- Packed with flavonoids, antioxidants and amino acid L-theanine
- Helps to produce germ fighting T cell(One kind of white blood cell)

Kiwi:

- Full of vitamin K, C, potassium, folate and essential nutrients
- Boost white blood cell to fight infection

Nuts:

- High in calcium, zinc and good fats
- Support immune system

Papaya:

- Loaded with vitamin C
- Have decent amount of potassium, vitamin B and folate
- Contain digestive enzyme papain
- Fight against inflammation

Pomegranate:

- Reduce viral infection

Poultry:

- High in vitamin B6 (Daily recommended amount of B6 -3 ounce poultry)
- Helps to formation of new healthy red blood cell
- Stock, broth contain gelatin, chondroitin and nutrients help in gut healing and immunity

Radish:

- Helps to regulate metabolism
- Boost immune system

Red bell peppers:

- Most vitamin C than any fruit or vegetable
- Rich in beta carotene
- Boost immune system
- helps maintain healthy eyes and skin

Shellfish:

(Lobster, mussels, crab, clams)

- Packed with zinc (Daily recommended amount of zinc -For adult men: 11 milligrams (mg), and for women: 8 mg.
- Helps in immune function

Spinach:

- Rich in vitamin C, numerous antioxidants and beta carotene
- Increase infection fighting ability
- Cook as little as possible

Sunflower seeds:

- Daily recommended amount -quarter cup serving
- Full of phosphorous, magnesium, and vitamin B-6 and E
- Helps to regulate and maintain immune system

Yogurt:

- Good source of vitamin D, calcium
- Helps in digestion
- Stimulate immune system to fight infection

Walnut:

- Boost immune system

Foods suppress Immune System:

- Alcohol:
    - Alcohol deprive body nutrition
    - Reduce number of white blood cells (fight against infection)
    - Excessive alcohol suppress the ability of white blood cells to multiply
    - Reduce killing ability of cancer cells

- Charcoal meat:
    - Any meat that is blackened is very bad for body
    - Cause infection
    - Break down collagen
    - Faster ageing process

Canned foods:

- Cans lined with bisphenol, which is suspected carcinogen (cause cancer) and   hormone disruptor which can weaken immune system
- Fried Foods:

  - Increase the bad cholesterol
  - Reduce immunity
  - fried foods accumulate acrylamide which is very dangerous for cancer

- Red meat:

  - Increase risk of cancer
  - Weaken the immune system

- Refined Grains

- Soda:

  - Interfere with body to get vitamin A, calcium and magnesium
  - Deplete calcium and magnesium in the body

- Sugar

  - Even small amount reduce white blood cell count (fight against infection)
  - Increase chance of infection

- Sugary snacks:

  - Increase attack of bacteria in the body

- Stop smoking

- Processed Foods (e.g. granola bars, dried fruits, margarine, flavored nuts, microwave popcorn, ketchup, frozen dinner, pizza etc)

Inflammation

Inflammation is a condition of the body in which a part of body becomes red, swollen, hot to touch and painful. e.g. arthritis, inflammatory bowel disease, vasculitis, pelvic inflammatory disease, rheumatoid arthritis, Diverticulitis etc.

Food helps to reduce inflammation:

Blueberries:

- High in antioxidants, phytochemicals and flavonoids
- Reduce inflammation in the bodies

Cumin

- Have anti inflammatory properties

Dates:

- High in fiber and iron
- Contain antioxidant
- Help to reduce inflammation

Dark chocolate/raw cocoa :

- Rich in antioxidants
- Dairy free 70% or higher reduce inflammation

Ginger:

- Have anti-inflammatory effect and help arthritis

Onions:

- Rich in antioxidants
- Have anti-inflammatory properties

Radish:

- Has anti inflammatory effects

Salmon:

- Loaded with omega 3 fatty acids, healthy fats and lots of nutrients
- Helps to reduce inflammation

Sweet Potatoes:

- Rich in beta carotene, antioxidants, vitamin C and B6
- Fight against inflammation

Walnut:

- Reduce inflammatory condition

Foods increase risk for inflammation:

Chips:

- Refined carbohydrate increase risk inflammation

Milk:

- Have affect on insulin, cause inflammation

See the food list that harm immune system

Irritable bowel Syndrome:

Irritable bowel syndrome is characterized by abdominal pain, bloating and alternative constipation and diarrhea

(Talk with your doctor /dietician)

Some important trigger factor other than food :

- Smoking
- Medications that contain codeine,
- Overuse of laxatives, and
- Depression

Some advices that are helpful for irritable bowel syndrome:

- Drink plenty of plain water every day.
- Drink water an hour before or after meal, not while eating
- Eat small
- Stop smoking
- Stop drinking alcohol

Food helps in irritable bowel syndrome

Cumin

- Helps to reduce bloating

Dried beans lentils, peas,

Flaxseeds

Psyllium husk

Soluble fiber (Oat, barley, brown rice, whole grain pasta ,Flesh of fruit, not skin, Dried fruit)

Soymilk and soy products

Foods should be avoid in irritable bowel syndrome

Alcohol

Bran (Insoluble fiber)

Broccoli

Cabbage

Caffine

Chocolate

Corn (Insoluble fiber)

Dairy products, especially cheese

Fatty food

Fried food

Large meal

Onion

Processed foods e.g. Chips, cookies

Refined grains

Soda

Kidney disease:

(your dietician may give you food chart with amount/limit)

Healthy foods in kidney disease:

Apple:

- Lower cholesterol
- Prevent constipation
- Fight against heart disease
- Decrease risk of cancer

Blueberries:

- Rich in vitamin C; manganese and fiber
- High in antioxidant phytonutrients called anthocyanidins,
- Contain sodium, potassium and phosphorus
- Reduce inflammation

Cabbage:

- High in vitamin K, C, fiber
- Good source of vitamin B6 and folic acid.
- Contain phytochemicals (usually found in fruits and vegetables) which fight against the cancer by breaking up free radicals before any damage to the body.
- Low in potassium.

Cauliflower:

- High in vitamin c
- Contain folate and fiber
- Full of indoles, glucosinolates and thiocyanates (helps liver to neutralize toxin)

Cherries:

- Contain antioxidants and phytochemicals

- Reduce inflammation
- Protective for heart

Cranberries:

- Contain Sodium, potassium, phosphorus
- protect against bladder infection (prevents bug from stocking to the bladder wall)
- Helps to protect stomach from ulcer causing bugs
- Protect against cancer and heart disease

Egg whites:

- Contain high protein, high sodium, high potassium and low phosphorus
- highest quality of protein with all the essential amino acids

Fish:

- Contain high quality protein
- Contain anti-inflammatory fats called omega-3s.
- Lower the bad cholesterol
- Protect against cancer and heart disease

Garlic:

- Reduce inflammation
- Lower cholesterol

Olive oil:

- Good source oleic acid (anti-inflammatory fatty acid)
- Rich in polyphenols and antioxidant
- Prevent inflammation and antioxidation
- Prevent heart disease and cancer

Onions:

- Rich in flavonoids (especially quercetin) which is an antioxidant
- Low in potassium and a good source of chromium,
- Helps in metabolism

Radish:

- Helps to wash out toxins from the kidney

Raspberries:

- Contain potassium, phosphorus
- contain a phytonutrient (ellagic acid), flavonoids (anthocyanins) and antioxidants
- Good source of manganese, vitamin C, fiber and folate, a B vitamin,
- Prevent cell damage by neutralizing free radicals
- reduce the chance of cancer

Red bell pepper:

- Excellent source of vitamin c and vitamin a
- Good source of vitamin b6, folic acid and fiber.
- Contain lycopene which is an antioxidant works against certain cancer and
- Low in potassium.

Red grapes:

- Contain potassium, sodium and phosphorus
- Contain flavonoids(Resveratrol)
- Prevent cancer and inflammation
- Protect against heart disease

Strawberries:

- Contain sodium, potassium and phosphorus
- Rich in phenols (anthocyanins and ellagitannins) and antioxidants
- Good source of vitamin C and manganese and fiber.
- Prevent heart disease
- Reduce inflammation
- Decrease cancer cell growth

You may have following foods in kidney disease : (Please always discuss with your doctors/dieticians)

Meat and alternative:

Food	One Serving per day
Beef, lamb, veal	30g (1 oz)
Poultry	30g (1 oz)
Fish , shrimp	30g (1 oz)
Salmon or tuna	1/4 cup
Cheese (hard cheeses such as cheddar, mozzarella, swiss, gouda, colby)	30g (1 oz)
Cottage cheese	1/4 Cup
Egg white	1
Unsalted Peanut butter	1 tablespoon
Tofu	1/4 Cup

Reference®http://www.hamiltonhealthsciences.ca/documents/Patient%20Education/Kidney DiseaseDiet-trh.pdf)

Milk and milk products

Food	One Serving per day
Skim, 1%, 2% or whole milk	1/2 cup
Cream (Half and half, light, or regular)	1/2 cup
Skim milk powder	1 and 1/2 tablespoons
Soy milk	1/2 cup
Cream Soups	3/4 cup
Yogurt, pudding	1/2 cup
Ice cream	3/4 cup

Reference®http://www.hamiltonhealthsciences.ca/documents/Patient%20Education/Kidney DiseaseDiet-trh.pdf)

Breads, Grains and other Starches

Food	One Serving per day
Pasta, rice(cooked)	1/2 cup
Bread	1 slice
Bagel, English muffin, pita	1/2
Cold or hot cereal	1/2 to 1/3 cup
Muffin or roll	1 small
Popcorn (unsalted)	2 cups
Crackers (unsalted)	6 to 8
Melba toast	4
Burger bun, hotdog bun, Kaiser roll	1/2

Reference:http://www.hamiltonhealthsciences.ca/documents/Patient%20Education/KidneyD iseaseDiet-trh.pdf

Foods should be avoid in kidney disease:

Artichoke

Avocado

Banana

Bok choy

Brussels Sprouts

Butter:

- Animal fat contains cholesterol, calories and high levels of saturated fat
- Margarine(from vegetable oil) contains trans fat

Buttermilk

Canned Food -Fish(Salmon/Sardines)/Beans/Lentils/Vegetables

Carrot juice

Coconut

Collards

Cheese-blue/feta/processed/processed cheese slices

Dates

Dried peas, beans and legumes

Eggnog

Figs

Fresh beets

Frozen meals/dinners:

- Most of the time heavily processed and microwaveable foods are high in salt, sugar and fat (e.g. pizza, cheese).

Guava

Granola

Grape fruit juice

Honeydew melon

Kiwi

Mango

Mushrooms

Mayonnaise:

- High in calories, high in saturated fat, high in salt and sugar

Okra

Olive

Orange or orange juice

Organ meat - Liver, heart, kidney

Oysters

Papaya

Passion fruit juice

Pear

Pumpkin

Peanut butter:

- High in potassium, limit intake (seek doctor's advice)

Persimmon

Pickles

Pomegranate

Potatoes

Powdered coffee creamer

Processed cheese

Processed cold cuts and winers

Processed deli meat:

- Significant source of sodium and nitrate which connected to cancer.

Prunes (Juice or dried)

Rapini

Rutabaga

Salt (Any kind of salt)

Salted nuts and seeds, salted snack foods e.g. salted cracker, salted popcorn, salted pretzels

Sauce (Barbeque, ketchup, mustard, chili, soy, steak, teriyaki)

Sauerkraut

Seasoned salt (e.g. chicken, garlic or onion salt and any food with salty seasoning e.g. prepackaged rice, potato chips and noodles)

Smoked or cured meat

Soda:

- No nutrient
- Packed with sugar

Spinach

Starches (commercial mixed of bread, muffins, cake, oatmeal, pancake, waffle, whole meal cereal, bran cereal, cornbread, salted pretzel sticks or rings, sandwich cookies)

Sweet potatoes and yams

Squash

Swiss card

Tomatoes

Vegetable juice/V8 Juice

Winter squash

Brain health

Beneficial foods for brain health:

Blueberries:

- May help protect the brain from some of aging effect.

Spinach:

- Contain powerful antioxidants
- Reduce the effect of ageing in brain function

Walnuts:

- Packed with omega 3 fatty acid
- Helps to protect against alzheimer's disease (memory problem)

Harmful foods for brain with ageing effect:

Applesauce

Bakery goods:

- Contain bad fat

Butter:

- Contain bad fat

Candies

Cane sugar

Chicken skin:

- Contain bad fat

Condiments

Corn chips, and

Corn syrup

Full fat dairy products :

- Regular intake has some effect on brain over time

Margarines:

- Contain trans fat bad for the brain

Potato

Processed baby food

Processed foods

Red meat:

- **Contain bad fat, has bad effect on brain**

Salad oils

Soda

Sugar syrup

Menopausal symptoms:

Food benefits in menopausal symptoms:

(Drink plenty of water according to weight)

Chickpeas:

- Rich in vitamin B6
- Helps to reducing menopausal symptoms

Complex carbohydrates:

- Brown grains, wholemeal pasta, bread and rice
- Helps to balance blood sugar level

Fresh fruits:

- Apple pears, grapes

Green vegetables:

- Celery, rhubarb and green beans.

Dates

Legumes

Maca powder:

- Helps with menopausal symptoms
- Reduce stress

Miso:

- Rich in amino acids

- Great for reducing cholesterol
- Helps in menopausal symptoms

Nuts

Oats

Raisins

Seeds:

- Pumpkin, sunflower, sesame, almonds seeds
- Prevent dry skin
- Normalize hormone level

Soya/tofu:

- High in calcium
- Easing menopausal symptoms

Turkey

Yogurt:

- High in calcium

Foods worse menopausal symptoms:

See the food list for premenstrual symptoms : Foods worse premenstrual symptoms and period

Premenstrual tension (PMT)

Foods helps to reduce Premenstrual Symptoms (PMS)

Artichokes

Banana

Broccoli

Brussels Sprouts

Chickpeas:

- Rich in vitamin B6
- Help reduce premenstrual tension

Chicken

Chia seeds

Eggs

Grilled salmon

Kale

Lean Beef

Miso:

Traditional Japanese seasoning made by fermenting soybeans with soy and koji (A fungi) or rice or barley.

- Rich in amino acids
- Great for reducing cholesterol
- Help to reduce premenstrual tension

Pumpkin seeds

Romaine

Spinach

Turkey

Quinoa

Wheat

Foods worse premenstrual symptoms and period

Canned food

Chocolate

Coffee:

- Caffeine increase boating and cramping

Dairy products:

- Cause cramping

Processed food:

- Package food, french fries, Chips, Dessert, fast food

Processed meat

Red meat:

- Contains arachidonic acid, which produces prostaglandins
- Cause uterine contractions and cramping

Salty food

Soft drinks/soda

Sugar

Spicy food

Refined grain:

- White Rice, White flour

Reproductive Health

Foods helpful for reproductive system:

Oysters:

- Contain more zinc than any other food
- Good source of proteins
- High in omega 3 fatty acids, potassium, magnesium and vitamin E.
- Helps in men's impotency.

Pink grapefruit:

- High in vitamin C and lycopene (carotinoid)
- Helps to protect from prostate gland disease

Pomegranate:

- Reduce the prostate cancer

Sleeping problem:

Some advices that might help in sleeping:

- ➢ Take the dinner at least 3 or 4 hours before you go to bed
- ➢ Don't take any heavy food/main meal/ dinner just before sleep time
- ➢ Elevate the head with 2 pillows
- ➢ Quit smoking
- ➢ Maintain a regular time

Foods help in sleeping

Almonds:

- Rich in magnesium, a mineral needed for quality sleep

Banana:

- Contain tryptophan help in sleeping

Cereal with milk:

- Carbohydrate and calcium, tryptophan in milk help sleeping

Cheese and crackers:

- Contain tryptophan and calcium , helps in sleeping

Dairy products:

- Contain tryptophan help in sleeping

Cherry juice:

- Boost melatonin level

Honey:

- Slight increase insulin that helps tryptophan to enter the brain

Hummus:
- Contain tryptophan

Kale:

- Loaded with calcium
- helps brain use tryptophan to form melatonin

Lettuce:
- Contain lactucarium, has sedative properties.

Pretzels:
- They have high glycemic index

Rice:
- High glycemic index

Shellfish:
- Good source of tryptophan

Tea (Chamomile/Passionfruit):

- Contain some chemicals that relax nerve and muscle

Tuna fish:
- High in vitamin B6
- Make melatonin and serotonin.

Walnut:
- Good source of tryptophan, a sleep-enhancing amino acid

Foods that harm sleeping

Alcohol:

- It may disturb your peaceful sleep

Caffeine:
- Even small amount of coffee can cause sleep disturbance
- Avoid caffeine sources, cola, tea, and decaffeinated coffee)

Dark chocolate:

- Even though it contain high antioxidant which is good for health, can contain high level of caffeine which can disturb sleep

Heavy food:
- Can cause uncomfortable
- Digestive system become slow during sleeping time

High fat foods:

- Hard to digest as digestive system become slow at sleeping time and disturb the sleep cycle
-

Spicy foods:

- Can cause heartburn and disrupt the sleep

Soda/Soft drinks/energy drinks:

- High in calorie

Stress

Food that reduce stress:

Asparagus:

- High folate
- keeps cool

Avocado:

- Rich in anti oxidants, lutein, beta carotene, vitamin E, B complex

Blueberries:

- Rich in vitamin C; manganese and fiber
- High in antioxidant phytonutrients called anthocyanidins,
- Contain sodium, potassium and phosphorus
- Reduce inflammation

Cashews:

- Rich in protein and fat
- helps to reduce stress

Dark chocolate:

- Dairy free 70% or higher elevates mood

Garlic:

- Good source of anti-oxidants
- Reduce stress

Grass fed beef:

- Source of antioxidants, vitamins A, C and E

Green leafy vegetables

Green tea:

- Helps to reduce stress

Oatmeal:

- Causes soothing feeling and helps to reduce stress

Oranges:

- Rich in vitamin C
- helps to reduce stress

Oysters:

- Packed with zinc which helps to reduce stress

Tea (Chamomile/Passionfruit):

- Contain some chemicals that relax nerve and muscle

Walnut:

- Omega 3 fatty acid keep blood pressure low
- Helps to relieve stress

Food that cause stress:

Caffeine:

- One of the cause of stress

French fries:

- Simple carbohydrate with trans fat cause stress, weight gain

Glazed doughnut:

- Added sugar increase stress

Granola bar:

- Added sugar, simple carbohydrate

Ice cream:

- Sugar causes stress

Nacho:

- Simple carbohydrate lift mood

Pretzels:

- Simple carbohydrate lift mood

Potato chips:

- Simple carbohydrate with trans fat cause stress, weight gain

Soda:

- Excessive sugar and calorie cause stress

Sugar:

- Any sugar causes stress

Urinary problem:

Foods that benefits in Urinary Problems:

Cranberries:

- Protect against urinary tract infections

Radish:

- It cleans out kidneys
- Inhibit infections in kidneys and urinary system
- Cure burning feeling during urination

Vitiligo

Foods are beneficial in Vitiligo:

(Helps to make melanin)

Almond

Apricots

Beet root

Bengal gram

Carrot

Chickpeas

Chilies

Copper glassful of water

Dates

Fenugreek

Figs

French beans

Green leafy vegetables

Jaggery

Mangoes

Onion

Onions

Pistachio

Potato

Pure ghee

Radish

Red peeper

Spinach

Walnut

Wheat

Whole grain

Foods can take once /twice a week in Vitiligo

Chocolate

Dairy products

Eggs

Ice cream

Milk

Poultry

Foods are harmful in vitilgo:

Acid foods (lime, lemon)

Alcohol

Blue berry

Cashew nut

Coffee, tea

Coloring agents,

Curd

Fast food/oily food, orange,

Fish

Garlic

Grapes

Guava

Palm

Papaya

Pears

Pickle

Pomegranate

Prune

Red meat

Soft drinks (Carbonated)

Sour food (tamarind, rhubarb, kombucha, gooseberry)

Spicy food

Sugar

Watermelon

Weight:

Some tips to maintain ideal weight:

- ➢ Take the dinner at least 3 or 4 hours before you go to bed
- ➢ Don't take any heavy food/main meal/ dinner just before sleep time
- ➢ Don't take large amount of food at a time
- ➢ Avoid high fat foods/fried foods and spicy foods
- ➢ Drink plenty of water

Healthy Foods help in weight loss:

Apple cider vinegar:

- Popular for dressing or vinegrettes

Almonds:

- Rich in the amino acid L-arginine
- Helps to burn more fat and carbohydrates

Avocado oil:

- Helps to reduce belly fat

Banana:

- Contain soluble fiber, makes feel full

Beans and legumes:

- Lentils, chickpea, black bean, kidney bean, soy bean, rice bean and others bean
- High in fiber and protein

Blueberries

- High fiber, low calories
- Helps to burn fat
- Flush toxins from the body

Brown rice:

- Rich in selenium ,manganese and antioxidants
- High in fibers
- Slow release sugar

Chia seeds:

- Good source of fiber
- Low in carbohydrates

Chili pepper:

- Contain capsaicin which helps to reduce appetite and increase fat burning

Coconut oil:

- High in good fats
- Increase calorie burn

Cottage cheese:

- High in protein, low in fat and carbohydrates

Cruciferous vegetables:

- Broccoli, brussels sprouts, cabbage and cauliflower
- High in fiber, low in energy

Chicken breast:

- High in protein
- Low in calorie

Fruits:

- Though high in sugar, low in calorie

Grapefruits:

- High in fiber, pectin helps to form bulky stools
- Rich in vitamin c
- Contain phytonutrients, fight against cancer
- Increase feelings of fullness

Green leafy vegetables:

- Kale, spinach, collard, swiss chards, lettuce, rapini etc
- Low in calories and carbohydrates
- Loaded with fiber

Green tea:

- Very high in antioxidants
- Thought to help fat burning

Lemon:

- A glass of lemon juice with warm water in the morning prevent fat deposition in the body

Oats:

- Packed with beta glucans and soluble fiber

Pomegranate:

- High in antioxidants
- lower the appetite
- flush the toxins from the body

Salmon:

- Loaded with high quality protein, healthy fats and many nutrients
- Can feel full for many hours

Tomato:

- Packed with vitamin C and lycopene
- Increase fat burning

Tuna:

- Low calorie, high protein food

Quinoa:

- High in fiber, nutrients, iron, copper, magnesium
- Contain all the essential amino acid to make a complete protein
- Reduce frequency of migraine
- Reduce risk high blood pressure and heart attack

Whole egg:

- High in protein, healthy fats, vitamins and minerals
- Low in calorie
- Egg in the breakfast benefits for weight loss
- Boost metabolism
- Make feel full

Full fat Yogurt:

Right amount can help to reduce weight (1 cup/day)

Healthy foods help in weight gain:

Avocados:
- Packed with vitamins and healthy fats
- Good food to gain weight

Cereal bars:

- Good source of carbohydrate
- May contain dried fruit, nuts or seeds

Cheese:
- High in calories and fats

Dark chocolate:

- Cocoa with 70% or more high in antioxidants, nutrient and calories

Dairy products:

- Rich of protein contain all essential amino acids for muscle growth

Dried fruit:

- Rich of high calories, antioxidants, fiber and lots of nutrients
- High in sugar

Full fat yogurt:

- Contain protein, carbohydrate and fat

Grain based cereals:

- Oats, granola, multi grains, bran, ezekiel are good choice for cereal
- Contain high antioxidants, fiber and other nutrients
- Good source of carbohydrates

Homemade protein smoothies:

- Can be made with milk/ almond milk with berry, banana, nuts or other fruits
- Homemade smoothies are always healthy

Milk:
- Rich in protein, carbohydrates and fats
- Packed with vitamins, minerals and calcium

Nuts and nut butters

- Very high in calories

Red meats:
- Best for muscle building
- Contain Leucine (amino acid), helps muscle building

Rice:
- High in calories and carbohydrates
- Digest easily

Salmon and oily fish:

- Excellent source of protein, healthy fats, omega 3 fatty acid

Starches :

Healthy starches are quinoa, oats, corn, buckwheat, potatoes, sweet potatoes, squash, winter root vegetables, beans, legumes

- add carbohydrates and calories to gain weight

Whole egg:

- High quality protein and healthy fats and nutrients

Whole grain bread:

- High in calories
- Good source of carbohydrates

Resources

Mclaughlin A, Foods That Suppress the Immune System, 2015,
http://www.livestrong.com/article/483356-foods-that-suppress-the-immune-system/

Carey E, 10 Processed Foods to Avoid, 2014, http://www.healthline.com/health/food-nutrition/processed-foods-to-avoid

https://www.davita.com/kidney-disease/diet-and-nutrition/lifestyle/top-15-healthy-foods-for-people-with-kidney-disease/e/5347

http://www.belmarrahealth.com/renal-diet-foods-eat-avoid-kidney-failure/

http://www.healthline.com/health/food-nutrition/foods-that-boost-the-immune-system

http://naturalon.com/top-12-things-killing-immune-system/view-all/

Ho J, 7 food that naturally fight eczema, CHATLAINE, 2016,
http://www.chatelaine.com/health/wellness/foods-to-eat-if-you-have-eczema/

Jung A, 16 Foods That Help You Sleep, Reader's digest,
http://www.rd.com/health/beauty/foods-that-help-you-sleep/

12 Foods That prevent wrinkles, BabaMail, http://www.babamail.com/content.aspx?emailid=13529

Foods that help or harm your sleep, Webmed, 2016, http://www.webmd.com/sleep-disorders/ss/slideshow-sleep-foods

Gardner A, Best and Worst Foods for Sleep, Health,
http://www.health.com/health/gallery/0,,20628881,00.html

Vitiligo Food & Diet , Ayurhealthline the herbal heritage of healing, https://www.ayurhealthline.com/Vitiligo-Food.html

L Jo, Eat to ease the menopause, goodfood Media brand of the year, https://www.bbcgoodfood.com/howto/guide/eat-beat-menopause

Kennedy Dr L, Top 10 Health Benefits of Brown Rice, Vegkitchen, http://www.vegkitchen.com/nutrition/brown-rice/

Bjarnadottir A, Why Eggs Are a Killer Weight Loss Food, Authority Nutrition, 2016, https://authoritynutrition.com/eggs-weight-loss-food/

Barnes Z, 6 Yogurt That Can Make You Gain Weight, Women'sHealth, 2014, http://www.womenshealthmag.com/weight-loss/eating-yogurt

Gragg M, 17 Superfoods That Fight Disease, Health, http://www.health.com/health/gallery/0,,20662664,00.html#yogurt-15

Wolff C, 7 Foods That May Make Your Period Worse, Because Nobody Wants More Cramps, Bustle, 2015, https://www.bustle.com/articles/99636-7-foods-that-may-make-your-period-worse-because-nobody-wants-more-cramps

20 Surprising Benefits Of Radish, Organic Facts, https://www.organicfacts.net/health-benefits/vegetable/health-benefits-of-radish.html

https://www.annmariegianni.com/5-foods-that-reduce-breakouts/

Glassman K, Mind Body Stress, Prevention, 2014, http://www.prevention.com/mind-body/emotional-health/13-healthy-foods-that-reduce-stress-and-depression

http://www.eatthis.com/foods-that-cause-heart-disease

Blumberg P O, 20 Foods That Age You 20 Years, EATTHIS,NOTHAT, http://www.eatthis.com/food-that-makes-you-age-faster